Ada

* * *

A novella about a sexy Texas lady

by T. F. Jackson, Jr.

1stBooks – rev. 05/23/01

Other books by the author:

* * *

Number 9

A memoir about growing up on a Northeast Arkansas
cotton plantation during the great depression.

* * *

Uncle Hot and Aunt Chur

He survived Iwo Jima.

She survived a vicious flashback.

* * *

'Lil Bit and Swift Eagle

A historical novel about cattle and sheep ranching
and the Comanche on the Western Texas frontier, 1868-1876.

Beginning of the End

Jake heard the fast approach and sudden stop of the pickup on the gravel in the driveway on the side of his house. He knew that it was Mike before he looked out, but he had to verify it. He was ready. He had known for some time that this day would come, and had dreaded it, but also seemed powerless to prevent it. But he was ready.

Hurried footsteps on the side porch.

Blam! Blam! Blam! Three not so gentle knocks on the kitchen door.

Jake opened the door. "Hi Mike .....

"Don't you 'Hi Mike' me you son-of-a-bitch!" Mike was storming into Jake's kitchen with the business end of a 12 gage pumpgun leading the way.

Jake acted undaunted. ..... "Come on in ....."

Jake appeared to look behind Mike, "..... you, too, Ada."

Mike turned to look back at Ada, wondering how the hell she had gotten there. She hadn't. Too late Mike realized he'd been had. When he had turned to look at Ada, he had swung the end of the shotgun barrel to the left of the intended target—

just far enough left that he would have to swing it back to the right to be on target. As he turned back to face Jake he found himself looking into the business end of a cocked .44 magnum leveled at his chest. He knew he didn't have the split second it would take to re-target—that by the time he swung the shotgun back to the right the impact of a .44 slug would have sent him backwards out the door and probably off the narrow porch into the yard with a hole in him the size of a grapefruit. He was smart enough and rational enough by this time not to try.

"Put down the shotgun, Mike ..... easy like ..... no sudden moves, or you're history."

The barrel of the .44 followed Mike's body as he slowly bent down to place the shotgun on the floor, and then followed it backup as he straightened up.

"Step inside and sit down at the table, Mike. Easy now ....."

Jake watched Mike move to the table—Mike seemed to be a bit dazed by the sudden turn of events. Slowly Jake bent down to pick up the shotgun, never taking his eyes or the cocked .44 off Mike. Quickly Jake worked the pump one-handed to eject the shell from the firing chamber, and continued until all the shells from the magazine were on the floor with the ejector locked in the open position. He released the ejector making a loud clang. Jake felt around on the floor to retrieve the shells, never taking his eyes or gun off Mike. He put the shells in his left front pocket and slid the shotgun down the hallway toward the utility area.

Jake then walked over to the wall phone, picked up the receiver and dialed a number, all with in his left hand. Jake's position was such that he could keep his eyes on Mike while he dialed. After the third ring there was a soft "Hello!"

"Ada?"

"Yes."

"Jake. You OK?"

"Yes."

"Mike is here. You better come over now. Come in the kitchen door."

"OK, I'll be there in a couple of minutes." She asked no questions or made any further comment. She hung-up.

Jake slowly replaced the receiver on the wall phone. He walked over toward the table where Mike sat, dejected, his hat brim covering his eyes that were looking down into his hands on the table in front of him, fingers interlaced, holding onto nothing. Instead of sitting down at the table, Jake pulled out a stool from under the breakfast counter, hung his left cheek on it, placed his left heel in the middle rung of the stool and extended his right leg straight out in front, all the time facing Mike. He laid the cocked .44 on the counter with-in the normal swing reach of his right hand, and sat looking at Mike. Neither said anything for what seemed like an eternity.

Jake's eyes wandered momentarily and surveyed the bright yellow with white trim kitchen. His eyes came back to Mike, but his mind thought about that first yellow with white trim kitchen that he and Marcie had. It had been a rather grungy apartment before they moved in. They had scoured off the many greasy layers that had cast a dingy pall over the kitchen walls, cabinets and ceiling, and then painted the walls a bright, clean yellow and trimmed the cabinets and woodwork in a gleaming white. The transformation was beautiful. The rest of the apartment was also cleaned and painted, but it was the kitchen that Jake remembered so fondly. When he moved into this house in Elmsville, he replicated the yellow with white trim motif of that early kitchen.

Jake knew that he should be thinking about the current situation—one that he had sworn he would never be in—but here he was. Mike was there at gunpoint, and Ada was on her way over. He had always known love triangles were the pits—especially when they involved someone else's wife. He should have a plan. He should know what he was going to do. He had no plan, and not a clue as to what to do next. He should be thinking on it, but that was too painful mentally. His mind drifted back to the happier time with Marcie in their small first apartment. Those were truly the "good old days."

Ada's soft knock on the kitchen door jerked Jake back to the present. He would have much preferred to remain in the distant past.

"Come on in, Ada, the door is not locked."

Ada entered the kitchen, looked at Mike sitting at the table, then at Jake slouching on the stool, and noted the cocked .44 lying on the counter. A sigh of momentary relief unconsciously escaped her lips. She had on no make-up. Her light brown hair with the hint of gray was pulled straight back and gathered by a bow at the base of her neck. She was wearing a bright, colorful house shift that fell from her shoulders with only the intrusion of her shapely breasts and their nipples breaking the downward flow of the garment. As had been her practice of late, she had on nothing under the shift. She was bare legged, and wore sandals on her feet.

As Ada stood there surveying the scene, the silence was so loud that it crescendoed, sending reverberating echoes through the minds of the three in the room.

Ada looked at Jake and said, "What gives?"

Jake responded, "I think he knows."

A soft "I know!" slipped from Mike's lips, his head still down turned, with his eyes looking at his hands.

"God ....." The unfinished exclamation from Ada hung in the air.

More silence, no one moved or said anything for some time. Finally Ada walked over to the table and started to take a seat opposite of Mike.

Jake broke the silence, "Before you sit down, Ada, why don't you put on a pot of coffee. I think we're going to be here for some time, and a cup of coffee will give us something to stare into and give us something to do with our hands."

Ada didn't respond, but went through the routine of putting on a pot of coffee. She didn't have to ask where anything was—she already knew. She sat down opposite Mike. The only audible sound in the room was the Mr. Coffee brewer bubbling boiling water over the ground coffee, and the made coffee draining into the pot below. Strangely the silence remained. None of the three seemed to want to start the talk, though each of them knew the talk was inevitable. The coffee finished making. Ada got up without any prompt and fixed the three cups of coffee, each prepared by force of habit to match the drinking taste of the individual—black for Mike, with cream and one-half of an artificial sweetener packet for Jake, and black with sugar for her. She slid the steaming coffee cups across the table toward their intended receivers. Jake came over and sat down at the end of the table, cradled the coffee cup in his large hands, and blew across the liquid's surface to cool it, as was his custom. He left the .44, still cocked, on the counter. Mike just stared into the coffee cup, making no move to pick it up or drink. Ada picked up her cup, and tentatively took a swallow—it was too hot, but she got it down.

Oddly it was Mike who started the talk with, "Well, where do we go from here?"

Jake came in with, "Are we sure where we are? We need to know that before we chart where we're going."

Ada looked first at Jake after that remark—a long deep penetrating look—and then turned to look at Mike. Jake had met her eyes and held them until she looked away.

Ada then got into the game of words. "I guess it's my turn. I'll start with where I think we are." She looked at Mike, and reached across and touched his cheek. "I'm sorry for the pain I may have caused you Mike, and may cause for you in the future. I'm also sorry for my own emotional pain, and ....." glancing at Jake, "any that may splatter on you, Jake. But I don't think we can get to where we're going without some pain."

"Before you go any further, let's think a bit on where we are so we don't go off half cocked," Jake said.

Ada

Where were they? That was a good question. Upon reflection, Ada realized that she hadn't really thought about that topic in depth. She had been taken up by the personal pleasure provided by the moment—albeit it had been a considerably long moment.

She thought back .....

She had grown up there in Elmsville, a small Central Texas town where you knew everyone and everyone knew you. Everyone also knew your business as well as who you were sleeping with, both routinely and any one night stands. It was hard to keep anything really private. There wasn't a hell of a lot of diversions in Elmsville, so as most small towns do, they made one of their own—being nosey and gossip. It was fun to talk among friends about the transgressions of the flesh, as long as they weren't yours.

She received her first taste of this dark side of small town life right after she had her first sexual experience. She was fifteen, he was Homer Wilson, and the place was the back of Homer's father's pick-up—a beat up old Chevy that ran most of the time. They had been to the local rodeo, taken a round about way back to her home, and the pick-up had stalled—at least that's what Homer had said. He had managed to roll it off the main road onto a field side road, where the mesquite brush conveniently concealed the presence of the truck. They had sat on the tailgate contemplating what to do, and filling in the thinking with a little necking. The necking got a little heavy, and before she had really thought through the situation, she was no longer a virgin. That first time was somewhat of a learning experience, and the results weren't very satisfactory, but they showed future promise. Miraculously, the truck started, and she got home without further incident, baring a little necking. She liked that Homer a lot.

That all turned to shit the next afternoon at school.

Becky Anderson, one of her big mouthed friends, sidled up to her and said, "You really didn't do it, did you?"

"Didn't do what?"

"You know, make out with Homer."

"Where did you hear that crap?"

"It's all over school. Homer was advertising it with the group of boys at the corner table by the window in the cafeteria at noon. I also heard it in the girl's john. A juicy tidbit like that spreads faster than a prairie fire in October."

"Shit! I'll never speak to that Homer again!"

"Then you did make out with him?"

"Shit no! He's lying!"

And that's the way it stayed for a couple of days. Ada decided not talking to Homer wasn't the best way out of the situation. She asked Homer to come by the house about 8:30 that night. Homer did.

Ada said she didn't want to go anywhere especially, why don't they just sit out in his truck for a bit. That was OK with Homer. She didn't get into the cab, but rather parked her rear end on the tailgate that Homer always kept at the horizontal to hold down on the drag. Homer slid over beside her, put his arm around her, and, since they were out of the line of sight of the front of the house, made a move to do a little necking.

Homer was then introduced to an Ada that he didn't know existed. She became much like the god of vengeance! He had on his football jacket, zipped up about half-way. Ada turned to him, moved her hands as if to put her arms around his neck, but instead grabbed the shoulders of the jacket at the collar close to the sides of his neck, and pulled down with all of her strength. The top of the jacket slipped down off his shoulders, pinning his arms to his side. It happened so fast that Homer was caught like a hog-tied calf. Ada reached down and unzipped his pants. Homer got out, "What the hell are you doing, Ada ..... ?" She reached into his crouch, got her a handful of balls, and squeezed as hard as she could. The effect was electric! Homer came off the tail gate, screaming with pain and jumping up and down. Ada came off the tailgate, too, staying right with him, maintaining a death grip on the balls. Homer went down on the ground, writhing in pain. It was only then that Ada let go. She then picked up a wrench from the back of the pick-up, put her foot down hard on Homer's Adam's apple, and spoke rather quietly. He listened with rapt attention.

"Damn you Homer, you son-of-a-bitch, you've been blabbing all over school about laying me the other night. Now here's the deal! You go back to school tomorrow and tell everyone that you were lying about laying me, and that we didn't make out."

About that moment Ada's father, attracted by the noise, stuck his head around the back of the house and asked Ada, "You'll OK?"

Ada responded without looking at her father, "Yeah Pa, everything is OK."

Her father went back around the rear of the house.

"Now, did you hear me Homer? Do you agree to stop this shit and tell everyone you were lying, or do I work you over with this wrench? On second thought, I won't hit you with the wrench. I'll just tear open the front of my dress and start screaming rape! How about that?"

Homer fully realized the consequences of that final threat. A few bumps and bruises from the wrench might be manageable, but Ada's six foot five, 250 pounds of old man thinking his daughter was being molested was entirely a different kettle of fish—dead fish! "OK, Ada! I'll do it! I'll tell everyone I lied! Now let me up so I can get the hell out of here."

"Promise?"

"Promise!"

She let him up and went back into the house before he could free his arms. She heard Homer's pick-up drive off.

"Ada's mom asked, "Homer leave already?"

"Yeah, Mom. He said he had some place he had to go."

Homer was as good as his word. He put out the word the next day that he had been fooling about having laid Ada, and that nothing had really happened.

The top of the day for Ada was when Becky came by and said, "Well, I guess you were telling the truth about not putting out any to Homer. Today he was telling everyone that he was lying the other day. He said nothing happened other than a little necking."

Ada responded, "You see, I told you that." Inwardly she smiled to herself. She thought, "Too bad about Homer. He had some possibilities, but his big mouth sure screwed that up." When she passed Homer in the hallway later in the day he avoided looking at her. Ada spoke anyway, "Hi Homer," and kept on trucking down the hallway.

The next incident that she remembered which reinforced the idea of not being able to get away with anything in a small town occurred a couple of years later. She and Oscar Small had a thing going and an understanding with each other about not seeing anyone else. There was a weekend dance and Oscar was out of town. She went stag along with a couple of her girl friends. There was an out-of-town boy—Billy Joe Conners—at the dance, and he was interesting to Ada. She danced with him a good bit, shared a couple of beers with him, and he drove her and her two friends home after the dance. He dropped off the friends first and Ada last. They just sat out in his car out in front of Ada's house and talked for a while, but he did walk her to the door and kiss her goodnight.

When Oscar got back in town the next week he came over to Ada's, and was mad as a boar hog with a sore tusk. He could hardly be civil long enough to get her out to his car. "What the hell went on between you and that Conners guy?" was the way he opened the conversation.

"Nothing. You weren't here, and he drove Doris, Becky and me home after the dance. That's it." She knew that wasn't the complete truth, but nothing had really happened.

"That ain't the way I hear it! It's all over town that you two made eyes at each other all during the dance, and that he took the others home first. You were out in the car with him in front of your house for a long time. What were you doing?"

"It wasn't a long time, and all we did was talk." Again, she knew she wasn't being real truthful. It was over an hour—her mother had come to the front window twice to see if they were visible sitting up in the car. They were.

"That ain't what I hear! You screw him?"

That tore it with Ada. "I didn't screw him! Take off Oscar, and don't come back! Damned if I'll put up such a jealous son-of-a-bitch as you are who won't believe me over some dirty, wrong gossip. Glad I found out early. Take a hike!" Ada got out, slammed the door of the car, and went back into the house. She would never have anything to do with Oscar after that, even though he tried hard to make amends. She knew that she hadn't been totally truthful with him, but she couldn't take the attitude of the question form of accusation that he threw at her.

After these two lessons Ada had been very careful about what she did and with whom she did it. She started asking herself, "What will the trouble makers say?" When she met Mike York it was good chemistry at the start. Mike was easy going, and didn't push where she didn't want to go. They were both ready to get married—everyone else their age either were married already or were frantically looking around for someone to do it with. It seemed the natural thing to say "Yes" when he asked her. She thought what she felt for him would last forever. They had had a good life together, at least for the first fifteen years. When their only son, Jimmy, was killed in an automobile accident it proved to be a turning point. Their personal affection for each other sort of drifted. They were still living together, but they didn't share much anymore. He had been partners with his dad in raising cattle, but they were over leveraged, and the bottomed out cattle market in 1973 started their slide into bankruptcy. The bank actually carried them for another ten years, hoping to get more money back from their continued operation than from a close-out. In the long run it was to no avail. Mike's father died in 1981. In 1983 Mike decided it wasn't worth the fight, and let the bank have the place. They were able to keep the house in town because of the Texas Homestead Act, but the ranch and cattle business went! Mike was able to get a job with the local feed, seed and fertilizer business as a representative that traveled the ranches and farms in the area. He had his job, and she had the house and a part-time job for her "beer money." They just seemed to go in different directions.

Ada was not a raving beauty. She was one of those women that had been moderately attractive as a teenager and in her early twenties, but seemed to improve with maturity. She had kept her trim shape, and her features, which were sharp in earlier years, softened as she matured. One of her attributes that fascinated Jake was her firm breasts. They didn't sag when "turned loose" and the nipples stuck straight out, like they were waiting for a nuzzle. She was pushing forty now, and looking better as time passed. Part of this was because she had learned how to accentuate her positive attributes and de-emphasize those that she considered to be less positive. The natural look became her, and she used it.

Ada originally had no intention of getting into an affair with Jake. That was the farthest thing from her mind, and if she had been asked, she would have truthfully responded, "Absolutely not!" When he moved in next door to her and Mike, Jake was just another friendly, older man. Albeit, he was a single older man, but that was of no particular interest to her then, either. He was nothing a happily married woman would go gaga over.

You could say that she wasn't a happily married woman at that point, but she was not unhappily married either. She wasn't hunting. It came on slowly. They had common interests in gardening, cooking, books, TV and movies, music, and more importantly, making love. She became aware of these common interests, gradually, over the period of a couple of years—and in that order.

It was their interest in gardening that got things started. Their gardens were side by side, and as they would happen to be working in them at the same time they would chat over the fence. Jake was much more into the technical side of gardening, and had a broader range in what he planted. It was his kitchen herb garden that got them together the first time in his place. They talked about herbs, she wanted to see his herb garden, he invited her over to see it, and he offered her a cup of coffee. She accepted and went into the kitchen with him. That was the first step toward their intimate relationship, although it didn't get down to the touchy-feeling stage for more than a year. When their relationship did get down to that stage, it was she who initiated the action.

Ada was really a warm, caring person who needed someone with whom to share her interests. The common interests that she and Mike had were centered on growing up in the same community and their son, Jimmy. After Jimmy died they had very little in common in the present and future. Mike was big on sports, hunting, and being one of the boys. Although she had an interest in sports earlier in life, it turned out that the interest was more in those male things that participated therein rather than the game itself. When she settled on a man, she lost interest in sports. She never was much into blood sports, even though her father had taught her how to shoot, as he had taught all of his children. She liked being good at shooting, but hadn't practiced much after she was married. Mike didn't have much time or patience with practice. He just wanted to do it—just like he made love.

As Ada had warmed to the budding idea of Jake as a romantic interest, she started to develop situations where they could be together. At first she insured that one or more of her female friends were with them when they were together. That was one way to put the quietus on any gossip about her and Jake, but bringing in a twosome or threesome to their meetings didn't last long. On one such occasion when Ada and two of her friends were at Jake's for a Chinese food cooking demonstration, her friend Becky asked Ada point blank if she had any proprietary interest in Jake. When Ada automatically lied, "No, not any," Becky smiled and said, "Then maybe I'll see if I can work up something."

Becky tried, but it was obvious Jake wasn't interested. Becky eventually got the message and focused her interest elsewhere. Ada would smile inwardly when she thought about it, but she quit having her friends around when she was with Jake.

Ada became aware that because of the physical location of their houses, it would be less noticeable to others for her to get in her car and drive around the block and park in Jake's carport. She could enter the carport from the back street that was rarely used by anyone. There were only a series of grown-up vacant lots on the other side of the back street, and the carport had a wall that screened off the view from the side street. She worked all of this out several months before she used it. Ada may appear to be devious with this advance planning, but she had some experience with the local gossip mill. If she ever decided to make a play for Jake, she wanted to be able to do it without Mike knowing about it.

To Jake it seemed that everytime he was working in his garden, Ada would be working in her's. At first he thought it was just coincidence. Later he concluded that it was part of a plan, but by then he liked the pleasure brought to him by the plan, and the idea that he had been "worked" into her plan was of no consequence to him.

Almost inevitably during the early days of their acquaintance they would wind up at the fence line talking gardening at first, and then branching out in many other areas. Jake decided that Ada was a very interesting person, one he would like to know much better. The fact that she was married kept him from overtly following up on this desire. Jake was not an overt home wrecker. It was counter to his basic character. Their eventual romantic involvement was delayed for some time by Jake's inclination to make no action that could be taken as an invitation, and to build nothing received into what could be an invitation. He did not play the role of pursuer, but rather he was more of an astute observer. This characteristic would have been discouraging to most females who had an interest in him, and at times it sorely tried Ada's patience. But Ada was both cautious and patient.

Ada had thought long and hard about what she really liked in Jake, and it came down to him being interested in her. Now this interest of his that attracted her was not just sexual, although he demonstrated a strong interest along this line once they initially got it on. He listened to her. She got back more than a noncommittal "uh huh" from behind a newspaper or over the blaring noise of the TV. He encouraged her to express her ideas on things and seemed to take a genuine interest in what she thought. When he countered her perceptions, it was in the form of a question such as, "What about so-and-so?" or "Have you considered so-and-so?" His approach to differences of opinion and perception were not confrontational, but rather the introduction of other material that, upon consideration, broadened her point of view.

The way Ada looked at it, the affair with Jake was a broadening experience. She got into it gradually over a two-year period. Like the frog in water where the temperature is constantly raised one degree every few minutes, she wasn't really conscious of the danger until she was already "cooked."

Even though she had the time to think out what she would do if Mike ever caught on, she had never faced that possibility in her "plan." Now it had to be faced!

Mike

"Where are we?" Mike thought, "Damned if I know." Since getting out of the cattle business, he hadn't had a care in the world. Today his world had gone to shit around his ears. He thought back about Ada. At first he had not noticed her. She was two years behind him in school, and that two years made a big difference until girls started turning into young ladies. When he had really first noticed her was when Homer Wilson was bragging what a good lay she was. Later Homer said he had just been lying to impress the boys, and he hadn't laid her. Mike still wasn't much interested, because at the time he and Mabel Kootz had a thing going. Mabel was a cheer leader and he was a big man on the football team. That lasted for about a year and they split. It was a couple of years later after he graduated from high school that he noticed Ada at a Saturday night dance. She was there with someone else and was having a good time. Mike was there stag and danced with her a couple of times. He decided she would be a fun date, and asked her to go with him to the next dance.

One thing led to another, and they got to be an item. She was a really good kisser, and liked to neck, but only so far would she go. There was a barrier that Mike just couldn't quite overcome. Every time he would think this is going to be the night, she would say "No" at the last minute. It always got him when she said that he was too special for a back seat quickie. Finally he figured that he would have to marry her to make out with her. He was right. He finally gave up and asked her to marry him. She said "Yes," and their early years together were absolutely fantastic from his point of view. Ada was all woman, and their sex life was great. They lived on his father's ranch for a while. After Billy came along they got their own place in town with the help of his dad for a down payment, but he still worked the ranch in partnership with his dad.

Billy was the center of their life. He was a good athlete, and was proficient at little league baseball and Pop Warner football. When he moved on into high school the coaches were glad to see him. He had done well as a freshman, and everyone was predicting great things for him in the future. Everyone thought he was a college level talent. Then came the automobile accident. A car full of kids out for a good time, a few beers, too much speed, and a sharp curve in the road—the car rolled over five or six times. Billy was DOA at the ER. Two other kids also died in the crash, and two were seriously injured. The sixth occupant, a girl, Janice White, was dazed, but otherwise unhurt. She wandered two miles to a house to get some help, but couldn't remember where the accident site was. They had to drive the roads in that area to find the accident site.

The whole town was devastated by the accident. No one was more crushed than was Mike. Ada hurt mightily, but she was strong emotionally. She spent her time comforting the other families that were involved, and spent a lot of time at the hospital with the two survivors. Mike needed her comfort, but couldn't communicate his need to her. Instead he walled off everyone and everything—he sought comfort in the bottle and solitude. The solitude was easy to come by, because Ada was busy helping others. She would check on him and he would say he was OK and for her to see after the others. She didn't have enough experience to know to do differently. They started to drift apart. It was a gradual drift, and for a long time neither was really aware of its depth or significance.

Everyone in Elmsville thought Mike was a nice guy. Everyone considered him to be basically honest—at least as honest as a good salesman could be. He didn't exaggerate the claims of what his agricultural products would do, although he might put the results in the best possible light. On a physical appearance basis, he was rather nondescript in a crowd, with no significant attributes that would make him stand out. He had an honest look about him, clean-shaven with a light five o'clock shadow. He was slightly above average height, and slightly heavier than average, with an indication of future baldness in the form of a bald spot that was gradually expanding on the back of his head. In other words, he was about as average looking as you can get for his age, just over forty. Being a Texan in the agricultural business, he normally wore modest western style clothes and good low-heeled boots. At home, he slouched around in a t-shirt, jeans and loafers. His vehicle of choice was a 4x4 Ford pickup, extended cab version. He knew it wasn't a necessity in his line of work—he stayed mostly on the paved roads—it was the image of the thing with the boys. He had persuaded Ada to get a Camero. He liked to drive it when the pickup was on the fritz.

Mike was a local football hero—one of the best defensive tackles to come out of Elmsville High, with the knack for sacking opposing quarterbacks at the most opportune moment. Unfortunately, he was just a bit small to be a college player, and he didn't have the patience to ride the bench for two or three years to get his slim chance at a starting role. He couldn't handle the adjustment from being a big player for a small school to being a small player for a college team that had many larger linemen who were just as quick, and with equal or better talent. He didn't have the heart to overcome better talent with determination. He dropped out of college midway through the first fall semester and returned to Elmsville to work with his dad. Everyone had expected him to make it as a college player, and his dropping out was a disappointment and an embarrassment to him.

He grew up on a ranch a few miles south of town. Everyone knew that the cattle business in which he and his father were partners went belly up in 1983. They had held on longer than most. The bank carried them because they were long time, trusted customers. It seemed to everyone who knew Mike, that he had lost heart for the cattle business after his father died.

Where they had been holding on by their fingernails before, Mike just let go and let the bank have it.

Mike didn't drink much after he got over the loss of Billy. He would have a beer now and then around the campfire at hunting camp, or with the boys during Monday Night Football, but that was about it. He was out on the road most days, so he only had an early breakfast and late supper at home routinely. In the mornings he would read the paper with a cup of coffee and follow up with a bowl of dry cereal—he didn't want to be bothered by a breakfast companion that talked. Many times when he had paperwork to do after returning to the office in the evening, he would call Ada and tell her he was going to eat out and work until he finished and for her not to fix supper for him. Ada had trouble trying to introduce him to a glass of wine with the supper meal. He would rather have a beer or a cup of coffee. Mike was a meat and potatoes type of eater. Ada found out that a quickly fixed frozen steak, micro waved baked potato, and a small green salad, followed by, or accompanied with, a large cup of hot, black coffee did the trick—every time. When Ada tried variations, substituting other food items, he would register a low-grade complaint by saying, "I like the steak and potato better." Dessert wasn't a big thing with him, and more often than not, it was rejected when offered.

On weekends during the hunting season he was out at the deer lease or the hunting club. He liked to talk about his hunting exploits, but since Ada didn't care for blood sports, she was not very attentive to his attempts at conversation on that subject. He found an audience with the boys. His prize trophy was the head of a sixteen point white tailed deer that was mounted on the wall of his den, above the shelf of his high school trophies. When he was at home, he was usually in the den, parked in front of the big screen TV, watching sports. He put in a satellite dish when he found out the wide variety and volume of sports shows that were available. He now had to make choices among conflicting sport events. He bought a VCR so he could tape conflicting sports events that he wanted to experience rather than read about in the local Gazette. When it came to reading, it was limited to agricultural trade magazines, Time, Sports Illustrated, and the popular biographies of current sports heroes by their ghost writers.

Ada didn't mind the satellite dish—it also brought in PBS, Discovery, A&E, and the movie channels. They were her cup of tea. She didn't much care for the soaps during the daytime—they depressed her because she could compare her own life with what was presented. She preferred intellectually broadening presentations, and occasionally a movie that would let her throw her mind out of gear and just float.

On the faithfulness attribute, Mike didn't have a perfect record, but he kept his hanky-panky out of town. There was a widow rancher customer on his route that liked for him to come by for a cup of coffee. Sometimes he stayed for half a day or more. There was also a divorced waitress over in Hopdale who was off work from 2:00-4:30 PM every day, and liked afternooners. Even one of the lady delivery coordinators, Della Burns, who worked with Mike had let him know she was available. Mike hadn't followed-up on this one, because he thought the advice "don't sleep with someone you work with" was very sound, yet he had to admit he was sorely tempted. He tried to keep delicate situations as far away from work and home as possible. Mike was not sex deprived, but rather enjoyed some variety on a rather discrete basis. Ada suspected because of how seldom Mike approached her, but made no investigation or inquiry because she did not want to know.

Now that Jake was around, she was happy to let her relations with Mike stay as they were.

Mike had found Jake to be a likable guy, but not his type. Jake could talk sports, but seemed to prefer not to. He knew a bit about guns, but was reluctant to talk on that subject for long. He was a bit too much into gardening for Mike's interest, but that was tolerable. Jake was an older fellow, and wasn't much interested in hunting, but did do a bit of fishing. Mike didn't like fishing. Jake's writing did not intrigue Mike, except for the diversity of the subject matter it included. Mike didn't understand how Jake could write so expertly on such a variety of subjects. Why didn't he concentrate in one area or related areas? Mike had trouble relating to the diversity that was apparent in some other people's lives. He was comfortable with the routine. The only thing in which Mike seemed to prefer variety was his sex life, and even then he stuck to a set of three partners.

Ada had introduced Mike to Jake soon after Jake had moved in next door to them. It was a Saturday afternoon. Mike was at home. The football game was just over, and Ada noticed that Jake was working out in his garden. She asked Mike if he had met the new neighbor. He hadn't. She suggested Mike go out and meet him. He tried to shy off with a remark like he would prefer for someone to introduce them. She said she could do that and before Mike could think of a good reason to stall further, she was out in the back yard yelling for Jake to come over to the fence to meet Mike. On another occasion she had invited Jake over for Sunday supper, so they got to know each other through her efforts. Mike and Jake had different interests, so their acquaintance stayed at the "How you doing," "just fine" level at a distance. Once Ada decided she had an interest in Jake, she no longer made any attempt to get them together.

Just last week Mike had overheard a conversation that he was not supposed to hear. He had walked into the local drug store, walked down to the end of an isle, saying "Hello" to a couple of older ladies along the way, and then came back up toward the front of the store on the back side of the isle. The conversation was between the two older women that he had passed on the other side of the isle. One woman said to the other, "That Mike York sure is a fine looking man. It's too bad his wife is cheating on him."

That picked up Mike's interest, and he listened hard, but the women shifted the conversation to a product they couldn't find on the shelf. He overheard no more on the subject of Ada cheating on him. He thought, "Who could Ada possibly be having an affair with?" He couldn't think of anyone right off that could be a likely candidate, and he knew about everyone in town. Perhaps it was only gossip with nothing behind it. But he would keep his ears open and stay attentive. He considered it unusual that one of his friends hadn't quietly said something to him if Ada was having an affair. Elmsville was a small town, and everybody knew everything about everybody.

It was a chance observation that convinced him that Ada was cheating on him with Jake. Because Jake was older, Mike hadn't previously considered him as a possible rival for Ada's affections. He had been blinded to that possibility by his own prejudice against older people.

Jake

"How did I get into this pile of shit?" Jake asked himself. It was a rhetorical question, because he knew damn well how he got there. Just like Adam, he hadn't been able to resist the forbidden fruit when it was offered, even though he knew that partaking would lead to his downfall eventually—if not actually, at least in his own self opinion. Being the outside intruder in a romantic triangle with a husband and wife was against all of his basic beliefs, but there he was, sitting at the table with the other two involved in the triangle—the meeting, now peaceful, arranged with the assistance of his .44 magnum. He came back to the question, Where are we now?" His mind wandered in contemplation .....

He and Marcie had been married forever it seemed. Her real name was Marsha, but her younger sister had trouble with that, and Marcie was how it came out. Marcie stuck. They were childhood sweethearts, starting from back in grade school. She was three years behind him in school, but she developed physically early, and in ways that attracted the interest of boys. They were an item so early in their lives that no one thought it would last. But it did. Like with every couple that dated for that many years, there were disagreements, some heated arguments, and momentary splits, but they got back together every time as soon as their tempers cooled. When they finally were married, a friend told them, "Well, you have known each other long enough that you ought to know what you're getting into." They thought so, too.

They were married when she graduated from high school, and it was a good marriage. She had agreed to work for a local institution for at least a year after she graduated, and Jake had volunteered for the Air Force rather than get drafted during the Korean War. They did some marriage commuting during that first year. Jake was sent to Lackland AFB in San Antonio for boot camp and then stayed on there, riding out his enlistment as permanent party. Their first year of married life was broken into a series of short periods—three day weekends and holidays—of blissful togetherness, followed by tearful separation, with many long letters bridging the time until glorious reunion, again tearful separation, and so on. Marcie had confided to a friend later that they had "set up and torn down housekeeping seven times during that first year." It was an ideal interlude when they finally got together for real. Neither had any idea how blissful being together full time could be. Before long the first of four bundles from heaven arrived, complicating their lives in some ways, but making them more fulfilled in others. Jeff, Jerry, Jonah, and Jason came along in that order over a period of ten years. Jake finished his four year enlistment, and then got a job as a writer, which was what he wanted to do all along—it was just delayed by the Korean War.

It was rough financially for the first few years—Air Force enlisted status didn't pay all that much, and the lower level writing positions didn't pay much better. Their married life finally became tolerable after the twelfth year, and then some easier about the time that Jason started to college. Jake showed some promise as a writer. He bounced around from one writing job to another across the country, trying to capture a living wage, and even had one overseas assignment to cover Europe for the syndicate for which he worked at the time. The boys enjoyed the European "holiday," but it placed a bit of additional stress on Marcie. She had worked until just before Jerry appeared on the scene, but she and Jake had decided it would be better for her to concentrate on being a mother, rather than go for the second income. It proved to be a wise choice. There was considerable self sacrifice on the part of Jake and Marcie while he worked up the economic ladder, but the results in the form of how the boys turned out as productive citizens were very gratifying. It was "worthwhile" was the adjective that Marcie had used. Jake struggled through the night school bit, finally getting a journalism degree—it took over ten years. After the boys moved out, Marcie went back to college to get a BS degree in American Studies. The boys scattered following their jobs, married, started families, and kept in touch by email, letter, phone, and occasional visits back home—which still kept moving about as Jake continued to change job locations. Everything was going well. Then it happened.

Marcie had been out interviewing for a job as a research assistant for a historian. When she came home she wasn't feeling well, and had a headache. She decided to just sleep it off. The next morning she was still had the headache and was listless. She laid around the house all day in her gown and robe. She could get some, but not total, relief from the headache with aspirin, but it persistently came back stronger after each medication. She said she didn't want to see a doctor just yet—she would go the next day if she wasn't any better by then. She wasn't. The doctor ran some preliminary tests, and arranged for her admission to St. Joseph's. She died that afternoon due to a severe brain aneurysm.

Jake was devastated. The boys all made it home for the funeral along with three of the wives and two grandchildren. Two days after the funeral Jake was alone for the first time in thirty five years. At first, he really didn't know what to do for himself. It had always been him and Marcie for as long as he could remember, and they had shared many interests. They had enjoyed sharing almost all of the little things that go with marriage, and the sudden absence of Marcie to share things with was very depressing to him. He would be doing something, a whimsical thing would happen, he would think, "I'll have to tell Marcie about this," only for the cold realization that Marcie wasn't there anymore to come crashing down on him. In talking about it later to the boys, Jake said, "It was one bitch of a time!"

Jake took the advice of the how-to books on survivorship in being a widower, making no significant changes in job or location for about six months. During this period the desire to change jobs and relocate kept growing in him until it crescendoed into an obsession. He had a little savings, and he decided to give up the slick magazine rat race and go independent. He also wanted to do some traveling—the wanderlust bug was at work something terrible. He sold the house, put some items in storage, held a series of going-out-of-fixed-housing garage sales, bought a pick-up truck and a small travel trailer, and hit the road. He kept Texas as his center of operations, but did wander into the campgrounds of the surrounding states. Generally he went north in the summer and was in South Texas in the winter. His experience with the northern US climate in his early working years gave him the inclination to head south in the winter—"anywhere south of Interstate 10" was the way he put it.

Using the contacts that had come with working in the writing game, he sold some special interest pieces and a series of articles for trailer traveling trade magazines. It was fun to get paid for writing about what you wanted to do anyway, although he had to admit he was no more than making bare living expenses. Some people wouldn't call his situation "living," but he was content. Then he got onto a nostalgia kick, writing two books for his grandchildren—their heritage from his family's point of view. Mostly they were about his early life and the family that he knew then. To his amazement, they sold, again doing little more than making expenses. He found a small publisher that specialized in those type books, and spent some time doing book autograph gigs, hyping his wares. Then came a couple of powder burners. He had always had a thing about western history, and more specifically the Texas frontier just before and after the Civil War. The sheep versus cattle ranching controversy intrigued him. So he did some research using the University of Texas libraries in Austin as primary sources of information. Again, these books got him on the road to author autograph sessions, and he enjoyed the exposure.

He liked the freedom provided by being an independent writer. He worked when he felt like it on subjects in which he had a great interest. Many times he would wake up at 4:00 in the morning, ready to write. A siesta in the middle of the day usually followed. Seldom did he routinely write after the end of the day, using the evening to read, relax and watch an occasional TV program or video. He really liked a good movie/video. He also found that being an independent writer had a problem side in the form of a broad interest that kindled many story ideas. His inclination was to follow a new idea rather than finish what was started on an older idea. He found his word processor cluttered with many starts and partially completed works, but few finished products. The deadlines of working for a publishing company provided both discipline to prevent procrastination and focus to finish off products. This was something that he would have to work on.

The trailer turned out to be a good interim solution for his housing problem. It served as home and office, and facilitated being mobile to pursue ideas and stories on location. The state of Texas had a lot of trailer parks in their recreation areas, and usually there was a river or lake there—a place for him to add evening fishing to his recreation routine. Long run, he figured he would buy a place and use the trailer for excursions, but that would take money.

It was during the powder-burner writing phase of his work that he decided he needed some diversity for personal recreation. The Whitte Museum in San Antonio was offering some Chinese cooking classes. He decided "Why not?" He liked Chinese food, and a little know how in one area had always lead him into some other interest. It happened here, too. The Chinese cooking went well, and dim sum—more specifically pot stickers—became his thing. This led to an interest in herbs, which reinforced the nostalgic itch he got early every spring to get dirt under his fingernails—the result of working the family vegetable garden as a kid. The trailer park in San Antonio had an area he could use to garden, so he did. The local Master Gardener group offered a training program, and he took advantage of the fourteen week Wednesday afternoon gardening school, paying back the opportunity by serving as a volunteer to support their school gardening programs.

All during this time he had no romantic interests, although he still noticed a well-developed front, a trim figure, and well shaped calves when they were in his vicinity. Marcie had said that when he quit looking he was of no use anyway. Marcie still walked with him in spirit, and he had gotten comfortable carrying on a conversation with her even though she wasn't there physically. Looking was OK. Touching was off limits! Those were her rules. This may seem weird, but it worked for him.

His disinclination toward romance was not because he was not attractive to the opposite sex or didn't have any charm. He was physically attractive, but even he admitted his charm, wit, and sense of humor were a bit off the wall. It had gotten him into trouble with Marcie on occasion. Once he brought home a large gift-wrapped box a few days before their anniversary, and told her not to bother it. Marcie could not figure out what could be in such a large box and be so light—she had picked it up and shaken it on the quiet. It turned out to be an empty box except for the note that said it contained his love and affection for her. Even though there was a real gift of a necklace, Marcie was a bit put out. She thought it should have been a larger box!

Another occasion that one of his presents got him in hot water with Marcie was a Christmas when the boys were all in their teen years. He gave Marcie two bright red pasties and a G-string. He just put it under the tree. Opening the gift in front of the boys embarrassed her. The boys all laughed and poked fun at her about the present. Although it pleased her that Jake thought of her as being attractive wearing the pasties and the G-string, she wasn't ready for the boys coming to that level of maturity. After all, a mother was supposed to be motherly and not a sex symbol. Behind closed doors with Jake, Marcie was as sexy as they come, but in front of her family, and in public, she was the model of motherly decorum.

Physically, Jake had taken care of himself fairly well. He was a few inches over six feet tall, somewhere in the range of two hundred thirty pounds, with rather handsome features. He had started balding from the front—a family trait. Only the graying of his hair tipped you off that he had topped the 60s hill. He grew a full beard when it became fashionable to have one. He went out of town on a writing assignment for a two-week period and returned with a close-cropped beard. Marcie decided she liked the beard, and it stayed. It also stayed closely cropped. Later it was modified it to a fu-man-chu. Because of his size, Jake was easy to spot in a crowd, but that is relative to the crowd. Once Marcie was to join him at a reception given by a pro basketball team about which he had done a feature article in the local Chamber of Commerce slick. Marcie couldn't find Jake for sometime. Jake said that it was the first time he ever talked to people's elbows.

Jake started writing short novels with a romantic twist—not the classic formula romance novels—but rather novels that had romance as a subtle ingredient. He never had a best seller, but their sales kept bread on the table. He noted his bank account also showed some prosperity. He had enough dinero squirreled away now in various savings accounts, CDs and other short term investments to buy a small place, and he decided to start looking.

Jake had a thing about serendipity. In his research for an article on today's trend in psychology, Jake had run across a journal article by Albert Bandura on the effect of chance occurrences in one's life. In effect, Bandura indicated that it was not the chance occurrence itself that would so significantly affect a person's life, but rather the individual's perception of the opportunity presented by the chance occurrence and the readiness of the individual—in terms of intellectual development—to take advantage of the presented opportunity. Bandura's concept closely paralleled Pasteur's position that chance seems to favor a person who is prepared for it. Jake had taken advantage of serendipitous occurrences to enrich the quality of his stories on many occasions. He was generally attuned to the opportunities that serendipity presented.

During one of his nomadic trips through central Texas he was pulling the trailer from one recreation area to another, when the pick-up broke down near Elmsville. He was towed in to the Ford place in Elmsville, and dropped the trailer off in a nearby mobile home park on the way. It took a few days to get the part in and fix the truck. During this time Jake rented an auto and spent some time driving around Elmsville. On one of his drives he came across a neat white house on a corner lot with a "For Sale" sign in the front yard. The house was plain, but neat, and it had a rear carport as well as a side driveway, and a lot of room for a garden. The garden area was grown up a bit, but the yard had been mowed and trimmed. There was only vacant land across the side road and the back road from the property. The house nextdoor look well maintained, as did the other houses along that street.

Jake decided to look into the price of the property. He liked the possibilities in what he saw. He jotted down the phone number of the real estate agent from the for sale sign. The price was right. Jake arranged to meet the agent at the house to see inside that afternoon. It was love at first sight—the house was just what he wanted. He laid some earnest money on the agent, and arranged to be back in a week to close. During the week he got his finances together and returned to close, paying $60,000 cash for the house and the two double sized lots that went with it. Jake took advantage of the serendipitous opportunity.

Prelude

The transfer truck arrived on schedule with the items that Jake had kept in storage for the past few years since selling the house he had shared with Marcie. Each item brought back memories as the truck was unloaded and the individual pieces of furniture were placed in the new house. The memories were bitter sweet—bitter because Marcie was not here to share the moment with him—sweet because of the pleasant memories of Marcie. That evening he just sat for a couple of hours in a big chair and stared at the furniture placed in the kitchen/family room of the house. The dimming twilight cast odd shadows that played tricks with his mind. He imagined Marcie was there and he talked to her. She was pleased with the house and his arrangement of their things in it. She was sure they would enjoy it here. He slept fitfully that night, extensively dreaming of Marcie for the first time in many months.

The next morning, after the first cup of coffee and before any breakfast, Jake went outside and walked around the front and side street property area. The house was white with a gray trim. Originally there had been two rooms across the front and one room that led off down the lot in a wing that was perpendicular to the front. A later addition had made a hallway down this back wing on the side next of the side street, and installed a bath on the opposite side as well as closing in a small bedroom. Still later an addition added a large kitchen/family room that extended into a utility area for washer, dryer, hot water heater, and a second bath with a walk-in shower. This addition ended at an outside door that opened to a large carport, wide enough for three cars—or a trailer and two cars—with a storage shed on the garden side. The carport was entered from the back street and had a wall that screened off the side street. The kitchen/family room had a fireplace on the wall opposite the side street, with the kitchen built-ins starting along the same wall about ten feet further on back. The built-ins included upper and lower cabinet units with a wide counter top on the lower units. A double sink with garbage disposal unit was under the wide window overlooking the garden. There were more cabinets and a large refrigerator that filled the remainder of the outside wall next to the garden. At the end of the kitchen the lower cabinet unit became a breakfast bar that turned out and then back toward the front of the house, making a "U" at the end of the kitchen. An electric wall oven was located next to the refrigerator on the side next to the double sink. A dishwasher was located under the wall oven. A stovetop was slightly recessed in the breakfast counter, extending some back into the kitchen open area. An overhead hooded exhaust unit was mounted over the stove top. There was a work table at the open end of the kitchen "U," that separated the kitchen from the family room part of the area. The work table was secured to the floor and had built in power plugs, with the wiring coming in through the floor and up one of the table legs. The effect of the breakfast counter was to restart the hallway, which had flowed from the front into the kitchen/family room area, back to the added shower and utility area and the door to the outside carport. The side street wall was actually a window wall across the length of the kitchen/family room area, with an outside door in the middle of the windows leading to a narrow side porch. There was a narrow gravel driveway that came off the side street near the front of the house, down beside the narrow porch, and then going back out to the side street. There were two large pecan trees on the back of the property—one between the carport and the side street—the other in the back area of the garden. The more Jake looked at the house, the more he liked it.

Jake went back inside the house, fixed a second cup of coffee, and then walked out into the garden area. He was mentally doing a layout for a small greenhouse, a compost area, raised garden beds, and considering what plants should go where. He noticed someone was kneeling down working on a flowerbed on the neighbor's side of the garden fence. He had been unaware of anyone being there because the person was screened from his view by the overgrown vegetation in his garden area. That was when he first met Ada.

The woman arose from working in the flowerbed and smiled. "You must be the new neighbor. I'm Ada York." She took off both of her gloves and offered her hand over the fence.

"Hi. I'm Jake Mechem, and I am the new neighbor." Jake took her hand intending to give it a polite shake. He was surprised that she gripped his hand decisively, giving a sound handshake from a man's perspective. He also noted that she had a wedding band and another ring on her left hand ring finger. He thought the other ring had a "stone big enough to choke a small horse."

Ada also noted his ring hand and that there was a wedding band on it. She asked, "Is your wife here yet?"

Jake was momentarily taken aback by this question, because he had gotten used to Marcie not being there, and considered everyone else had, too. Then he realized that he still wore his wedding ring. He smiled. "No, there is no Mrs. Mechem now. Marcie died some time ago. I still wear the ring from force of habit."

She responded, "That's touching."

After a moment of silence she moved on with, "I'm glad someone is moving in. I hope you can do something with the stuff growing up in this garden area."

"Yes, I'm going to do something about the garden. It's time to start the fall garden, and I'll get it cleared out this week. Is there a nursery in town that sells gardening supplies and transplants?"

Ada told him where the places were in town that sold plants, seed, and out door tools. That was their initial meeting—the first of many more to come.

Ada watched with interest while Jake turned the overgrown weed patch into a model garden—at least a model in Jake's eyes. The garden area was as big as most city lots. He was partial to raised beds, drip irrigation, compost piles, and even organic gardening, to a certain degree. He was no purist, and pesticides were part of his armamentarium, but he preferred to use natural pest controls when practical. He also was not a vegetable garden purist in that he included cut flowers, color beds, fruit bearing vines, and small fruit trees along with the traditional vegetables. He liked to do a lot of experimenting with various types and varieties of plants, working to find out what produced best in this particular area.

Jake installed a small prefabricated greenhouse next to the carport storage shed on the garden side of the property. He also had a load of topsoil and old railroad ties hauled in, and he established a series of compost piles near the greenhouse and by the large pecan tree. He cut the taller weeds with a brush hook, and then ran them through a shredder.

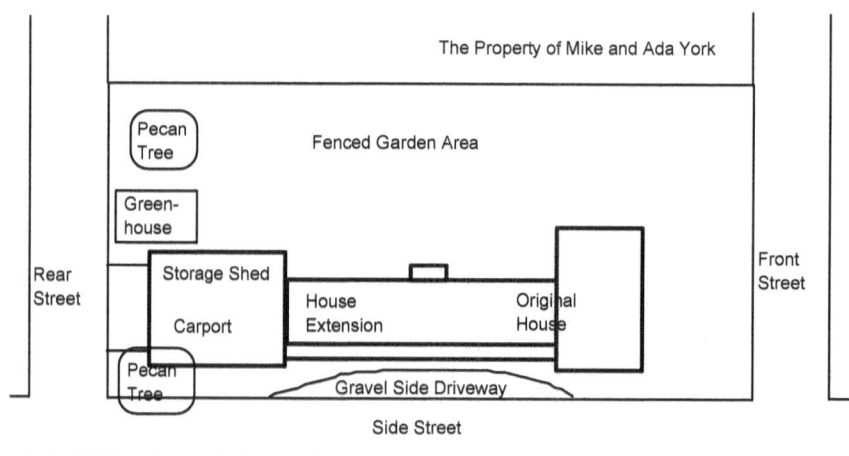

Plot plan of Jake's property.

to turn them into material for mulch. Then he used the compost setting on the lawn mower and cut and bagged the rest of the weeds, adding them to the compost piles. Ada watched the operation from across the fence with more than mild interest. She thought, "That looks like a pro at work."

Since it was mid-summer, and time to start the fall garden, Jake established six four-by-eight raised beds toward the back of the garden, leaving the rest to be put in for the next spring garden. He kept the rest of the area mowed through the end of that fall gardening season, using the clippings for compost. As the weather cooled, the fall garden really came on strong. As the tomatoes and vegetables matured, Jake offered some of them to Ada from time to time—the Yorks hadn't put in a fall garden, and their plants were down to the nonproductive stage. Once a killing frost occurred, Jake removed all the old plants and composted them. He then planted Elbon rye grass in the growing areas to control nematodes and provide organic material for the next growing season.

Ada spent a lot of time during the next few months at the fence line talking to Jake about what he was doing in the garden. Jake was glad to have a neighbor that was interested in his gardening, and was free with conversation, information and gardening advice. He had met Mike, and noted that Mike did not share Ada's enthusiasm for gardening, although he seemed to like for Ada to be into gardening—"gives her something productive to do." On many occasions Ada would bring two cups of coffee out to the fence line, pass one over to Jake, and they would share a few moments in conversation. Several times Jake invited Ada over so she could see up close what he was doing in the rear of the garden area—the new plants in the greenhouse, the composting operation, and some new dwarf fruit trees he was starting. On these occasions he would offer her a cup of coffee, and she usually accepted. At first they shared the coffee and conversation outside in the back part of the garden where Jake had set up an A-frame mounted swing. Then from time-to-time she would go into the house and share the coffee in the kitchen/family room area—sometimes at the counter, sometimes at the worktable, and sometimes in front of the fireplace area. She really liked the fireplace area in the winter when Jake had a fire going. Jake didn't use the worktable so much as a kitchen worktable, but rather had four chairs placed around it. Most of the time they sat at the worktable to drink coffee and talk.

Over time they found out they had many mutual interests. They both liked good movies, especially ones that would let you turn your mind off and float. Jake tended to like action movies more than did Ada. She tended to go for the man-woman relationship movies that worked out right in the end. Both liked PBS, Discovery, and A&E channel documentaries and information programs. The CNN channel news programs were also a common interest. CNN let you have the news when you wanted it rather than only at 6:00 and 10:00 when the networks scheduled to dish it out. On several occasions when there were fast breaking major news stories they would spend some time following events as they occurred—such as the California earthquakes near where one of Jake's boys lived.

Jake found out that Ada also liked out-of-doors activities. She just didn't like to hunt with Mike because he made a big thing out of it rather than just recreation. Neither did she care for being with "the boys" that Mike ran with. She liked to hike, picnic, and could put up with fishing. Sports were not of much interest to either of them, although Jake sometimes watched parts of pro baseball, football and basketball games. Many times he would deliberately catch only the last few minutes of a game—that time period contained the most exciting parts of the game, and he got the final score.

Ada grew to like the way Jake did things. He never talked down at her, and always treated dumb questions with a respectful response. He had the knack of breaking down a complicated idea into understandable parts that lead to an explanation, yet he did not seem to oversimplify its complexity. As the Elmsville people found out they had a professional writer in their midst, they began to offer invitations for Jake to speak at various civic and public gatherings, usually to either talk about writing in general or a subject upon which he had written. Jake enjoyed talking to the local high school journalism classes, and the local garden club. He tended to shy away from lady's club meetings unless the subject was a specific book he had written. You had to do what you had to do to sell books, but ladies club activities generally bored him sick. Ada kept up with the places that Jake was going to give presentations, and where it wasn't so obvious for her to do so, she usually arranged to attend. She made it a point to stay away from Jake during these affairs, allowing Jake to spend time with others, and she usually left as soon as it was proper to leave.

Ada realized that she was becoming strongly attracted to Jake romantically, but tried desperately not to let it show to anyone but Jake, and even very gradually and carefully to Jake. She knew the town and what its wagging tongues could do. Jake never made a play for Ada. That was not his style. Married women were off limits, and he hadn't seen any unmarried women that turned him on—loyalty to Marcie was still very much in evidence. Jake seemed to ignore the subtle pitches that Ada would make—those that could mean nothing, or could lead on to something, depending on how they were taken and the return response. Every time Ada would step up the intensity of her subtle approach, Jake would go out of town to visit his publisher or for a book signing engagement. Jake played everything straight down the fairway, demonstrating no inclination for hanky-panky out in the rough. Ada was getting frustrated. Jake was getting frustrated with the situation, also. He liked Ada much more than he would admit. He recognized the subtle invitations from Ada, and had so far been able to ignore or turn them harmlessly without increasing the intensity of their involvement. He wanted to maintain their current relationship, and not raise the intensity to a level that would eventually lead to them having to break it off. He enjoyed her company very much. If she weren't married to Mike, Jake would have long ago made a play for her intimate affections.

That was how things rocked along for almost two years. Jake and Ada spent a lot of time together sharing their common interest in gardening and things in general. Ada kept up the subtle pressure, and Jake deflected each of her subtle approaches with great skill—against a growing inner desire for her that was approaching an obsession, an obsession to which he didn't think his conscience would allow him to surrender.

Entrapment

Jake caught a rather severe cold the second winter that he lived in Elmsville. This created the situation in which Jake and Ada ignored the obvious problems involved with the trend of their relationship, and went for it.

Because of his cold, Jake stayed inside, and didn't work in the garden area for a couple of days as he usually did, even though the weather on those days was warm and fair. His absence from his usual haunts was noted by Ada, and she called him on the phone. She said she would bring over some chicken soup—her traditional family treatment regimen for recovery from a cold. He said he would leave the kitchen door unlocked. She asked him to leave the carport door open instead. He did.

Ada arrived, bright and bubbly, with a crock of hot chicken and vegetable soup and a bouquet of fresh cut flowers. Jake was lying on a day-bed type of couch in the family room area, propped up on a pile of pillows, and dressed in a set of unmatched sweats. He kicked off the Afghan that was covering him, sat up, swung his feet to the floor, and started to find his slippers.

63

Ada said, "Don't get up. I know where things are, and I can manage. Lie back down and rest. Everything is under control. Doctor Ada is here!"

Jake laid back down. He watcher her with admiring eyes. She was a smooth flow of color in the bright shift as she glided around the kitchen. She put the crock in the microwave to re-warm the soup, and then retrieved a vase from one of the bottom cabinets. She made a fuss about arranging the flowers in the vase and then placed them on the table at the end of the couch so Jake could admire them. The microwave alarm sounded to indicate the soup was warmed, and she took two bowls from the dish cabinet. She kept up a line of light banter while she was doing these things, the type of banter that requires no response. Jake didn't respond—just watched her perform with bright eyes and a smile. She ladled the soup into the two bowls, located two soupspoons and paper napkins, and moved toward Jake.

"Jake, do you want anything to drink with the soup?"

"No. Nothing. No crackers and nothing to drink." Jake raised himself up and swung his feet to the floor, accepted the soup and accessories, and tasted the soup. Too soon! The soup was too hot, and it burned his mouth.

Jake exclaimed, "Damn! You must have warmed it twice!" He put the soup on the magazine table in front of the couch. "That will have to wait a few minutes to cool off."

Ada placed her soup on the magazine table. "While we're waiting for the soup to cool, I'll give you a back rub. Lie down on your stomach."

Jake started to protest, but she took a bottle of lotion from her handbag, crossed the room, and pushed him down on the couch. "On your stomach! Doctor's orders!"

Jake complied.

Ada pushed up his sweat shirt, poured some lotion on her hands, and began to massage his back. She knew how to give a back-rub. Her strong hands and long fingers applied just the right amount of pressure and rhythmically stroked his back, top to bottom. Her fingers dug deep into his back muscles, causing them to relax.

Jake's back hadn't felt this good in a long time. "You give a right fine back-rub doctor. How much do you charge?"

"You can't afford me. Turn over."

Jack automatically complied, and what happened next was outside of his expectation. Ada had poured more lotion on her hands and rubbed them together. Then she slipped her right hand under the front of his sweat pants and began to gently caress that area. Jake started to raise upright, but she pushed him back down with her free hand.

"What are you doing, Ada?"

Ada turned a set of soft, misty brown eyes toward his face and whispered, "If you don't know, I must not be doing it very well."

Jake knew! It didn't take an Einstein IQ level to figure that out.

"Ada, it's been so long since I had a woman that I don't truthfully know whether or not the equipment will work."

Ada could tell by the response to her touch that the equipment was going to work just fine.

Jake continued, "You know that we shouldn't be doing this?" It wasn't really a question, but a half-hearted effort to climb away from the abyss toward which they were rapidly sliding. Half of him ached for the sexual pleasure that he knew could come from this affair, but the other half hesitated because of the potential dire consequences of partaking of forbidden fruit.

Ada kissed Jake like he hadn't been kissed for a terribly long time. "Shut up Jake, and make love with me." She stood up and took the shift off over her head. As Jake had suspected, she wasn't wearing anything under the shift. The sight of her well-sculptured form blew away all of Jake's rational resistance. "God, she's beautiful," Jake thought—his current sexual desire might have influenced his judgment here.

Ada reached down and slipped off Jake's sweat pants, and then sat astride of his loins, placing her knees up along side of his chest with her lower legs and feet folded back. It was an instant fit. The equipment seemed to know what to do, and responded automatically. Jake forgot about being sick.

Jake slid his hands up the sides of her stomach, up to those beautiful, well formed breasts with the protruding nipples, and softly caressed them, cupping them into his hands. Ada began a rhythmic bump and grind motion with her torso. He responded stroke for stroke. He raised himself up on his elbows, and nuzzled her nipples with his lips. He began a soft sucking of the nipples, and she responded by pushing her breasts toward him, without changing her pelvic motion. They remained in this ecstasy for much longer than Jake had expected. He had thought he would explode instantly with contact, but the equipment worked well, and resisted climax until Ada's breathing and the increased rapidity of her contortions indicated she was there—they went together. They remained in that position for several minutes, she with her eyes closed and tongue wetting her lips, and he lying back, relaxed.

Without getting up, she bent over and reached down on the floor to her purse and extracted a handful of tissues. She shared them with Jake, and then straightened out her legs and slid down beside him on his right. He held her and she held him. She snuggled down on his shoulder, burying her face in his neck. They remained in this position for some time, neither talking, both quietly enjoying the afterglow. They fell asleep like innocents. It had been fantastic, better even than either of them had imagined that it could be.

Jake didn't know how long they had been there like that. He awoke with a start. The phone rang. He settled back realizing the answering machine would handle the call. Ada just snuggled closer to him. He reached over and spread the Afghan over them, and they drifted back to blissful sleep, ignoring any pending danger that could come from their current position. The call was from his publisher, and was of no immediate consequence.

Sometime later Jake awoke, but remained lying there motionless, relishing the feel of Ada next to him. She stirred, and he kissed her lightly.

"You can do better than that," she said, and then hung a long passionate kiss on him.

"My cold ..... ," Jake offered.

"Your cold is the least of my worries, Jake Mechem," she responded, and kissed him again. Jake kissed her back.

Eventually she got up, picked up her shift, slipped into her sandals, started walking toward the bath in the utility area, and said over her shoulder, "I need a shower. Do you have any shampoo? You want to come along with me? I'll let you wash my back."

"Can I wash your front?" Jake asked.

"Come along and find out."

He did and he did. Jake hadn't had sex on the hard surface of a shower's tiled floor in a long time, but it was just as good as he remembered it. He didn't even mind being on the bottom. That was one of Ada's conditions. Later she said, "I should have made you provide knee pads, too." Jake decided that he would have worked something out if she had asked. Jake was also amazed at his newly found sexual endurance. It hadn't always been that way. He was looking back at sixty, hadn't been screwed during the five years since Marcie's death, and he had performed well twice within a couple of hours. He expressed his thoughts honestly to Ada, indicating some wonder at what had happened. She responded with, "You just needed the right inspiration." Jake liked very much what he had experienced of the inspiration. He countered with, "Keep up the good work, Doctor!"

It was a miserable, cold, wet winter day outside, but it was a warm spring day filled with sunshine inside. They dressed after the shower, and Ada reheated the soup. They sat at the kitchen table and ate. Jake really liked the soup, and said so, "This is really good soup. You're a good soup fixer, Ada."

"I bet you tell that to all the women that you seduce," Ada responded.

Jake just kept eating and let that remark lay there. He thought she seduced him. A few moments later he broached the subject he dreaded. "What about Mike?"

Ada responded, "What about him?" She went on with, "Mike won't be in until another two-three hours. Supper fixings are in place. It's no problem." She could tell by the look on his face that her response hadn't helped their situation any. She continued, "If you mean 'Am I going to tell him about this?' hell no. This is too good of a thing to let him mess up, and I want to continue with this in the future ..... if you also would like to continue, of course. We just need to be careful, and not be seen out in public together. Mike has other interests. He won't be much of a problem."

- - -

Sitting at the table now with Ada and Mike, Jake thought that Mike could easily turn out to be a much bigger problem than either he or Ada had bargained for. Mike had been extremely agitated, but was quiet and reflective now. Jake wondered, "What would have been the outcome if he hadn't been ready for Mike. What would have happened if Mike had just come in firing that pump-gun and not talking? What if Mike had used the pump-gun on Ada before coming after him?" There were many possible alternative happenings other than what had taken place. So far, the Lord had smiled upon them. Jake just hoped He didn't change His mind.

Deception

The deception of Mike was the norm for Jake and Ada during the next year or so. Jake found out that Mike had a routine schedule that seldom varied, and when it did vary, Ada knew about it in advance. The ease with which Mike could be deceived made Jake and Ada a little over sure of themselves as the affair continued. It required little discipline—just play it straight when Mike was around, and don't be seen together in public when he wasn't.

It is not accurate to say that Jake and Ada callously kept the affair going with a total disregard for Mike. The problem of their romantic triangle was much on their minds and the topic of their conversation many times. Jake had a guilty conscience and avoided Mike whenever possible. He talked to Marcie about the affair on numerous occasions, but she didn't seem to provide him any real answers. In his mind's eye she just sat and looked at him as he poured out his guilt and doubts. She had done this somewhat during her life. When he had a problem, he would lay it out for her. She would listen patiently, and then give him that look that meant, "It's your problem—you fix it."

Just talking things through to her had usually been helpful then, giving him a more complete perspective of the problem's ramifications. In this particular situation, it wasn't helping. He still had a subconscious loyalty to Marcie, and the act of talking to her about the affair only raised his guilt complex. Jake couldn't come up with a way out where everybody won, and he could come up with many possible scenarios that got his ass killed. At the same time, the thought of life without Ada was very painful to him. Maybe some problems just naturally don't have win-win solutions, and truly have only distinct winners and losers. At numerous times Jake would decide the affair should be ended, but at the sight of Ada, his resolve melted away, pushed from his thoughts by his genuine love for her and the burning desire to be near her. It was not just a sexual attraction. It was much more. It included wanting to be with her all of the time, and sharing the little things of life. It hurt every time she left him to go back to her married world and Mike.

Ada and Mike shared many common bonds from the past. Most important of these was the memory of Jimmie. Their memory of him was both a part of the glue that had held their fragile marriage together to this point, and also a factor in its deterioration—at least their reactions to his untimely death were. As is usual among long term married people, they knew the habits, likes, and dislikes of each other, and to an extent, each generally catered to the known desires of the other. At least they didn't deliberately go out of their way to piss each other off, and for the most part they actively worked at making the routine of life pleasant for each other, if it didn't interfere with what they wanted to do. Ada though it was a real tragedy that her marriage, which had such a good beginning, would degenerate into little more than peaceful coexistence with each of them going their own way.

The routine that Jake and Ada settled into with the affair was rather simple. They were together in a lover's relationship only in his house. She would drive up the back street and park in the carport, entering through the back door. Jake had an extra key made for her so she could come and go at will. Mike was out of town for at least six hours every day during the week, working the contacts on his sales route. On the week days Ada wasn't working—she worked two days a week as a fill-in cashier at Walmart—she would come over to Jake's place midmorning, after calling Jake to make sure it was OK for that day. They would have lunch, taking turns cooking for each other, while the one not cooking would sit across the breakfast counter and kibitz. They didn't always make love every day during her stay, but most of the time they did. Sometimes they make love more than once—on a few days even as many as three times. They just let it happen, whenever they felt the desire. There was a very strong mutual physical attraction, and it didn't take much to turn either of them on—sometimes it happened at first sight, just by being there.

On weekends it proved to be catch-as-catch-can. If Mike was off on a hunting trip, Jake and Ada would usually get together Saturday morning and spend the day together. On the times Mike went some distance away to hunt, she would spend Saturday night with Jake. When that happened she was always careful to return the Camero to her driveway, and walk over to Jake's via a back gate to her garden and along the back street, coming in through the carport as usual. Jake and Ada would experiment with gourmet cooking, have late night refrigerator raids, dance, watch TV if it was a good programming night, share a video, or just read—and make love—sometimes on the couch, in the floor in front of the fire place, with her sitting on the lower kitchen cabinet or work table, in the shower, and in bed. Jake had a small video collection, and sometimes he would pick up a current popular video from the video store. Sometimes they never got around to watching the video. In the morning they would share coffee while propped up in bed on a pile of pillows, and get a handle on what was going on in the rest of the world with CNN. Being together on these mornings after would also frequently develop into love making sessions. They had trouble keeping their hands off each other when they were together, and they responded to each other's touch—it was mutual.

Those over-nighters made Jake hungry with the desire to be with her all of the time, but he couldn't work out just how to do that yet. Ada had openly expressed the same sentiment once to Jake as she was snuggled into his shoulder on a Saturday night, "Jake, I would like for it to be like this all of the time. I like it here at night. It feels comfortable and warm and safe. I don't want to go home." Jake didn't say anything then, but held her tightly. He quietly thought, "I would like to be with you all of the time, too, but I don't relish the idea of Mike going hunting at my house with me providing the trophy. My head wouldn't look near as good on his den wall at that sixteen point buck." Ada did go home the next day, without again bringing up the subject of staying at Jake's full time.

As spring came on, both Jake and Ada worked in their gardens, frequently side by side, and openly shared refreshments outside in the yard at both houses. Mike and Ada had a back patio that was shaded, and Ada would invite Jake over for lemonade or iced tea and cookies. She never invited Jake inside. Jake likewise would invite Ada for refreshments, and serve them out by the A-frame swing. Ada liked that swing. They kept these type meetings public because they were natural among friendly neighbors. Ada would mix in talk of Jake's garden, their common garden interests, and some of their working together on gardening projects, and even her going over to see parts of Jake's garden and having a cold drink in her conversations with Mike, who appeared to be comfortable with the relations between them and their next door neighbor. He said something to Ada once to the effect that she hadn't invited Jake over for some time. She responded, "I didn't think you two shared many of the same interests, and I didn't want to saddle you with a boring guest. I'll invite him over if you would like for me to." Mike indicated, "Don't bother. You're right, we don't have much in common." That was fine with Ada. She preferred they not be too close now.

Jake's productivity as a writer suffered some in quantity because of the amount of time he spent with Ada, but the balance of improved quality was enough to keep him out of trouble with his publisher. Ada seemed to turn on his creative talent, and his writing improved—not so many extensive rewrites or blockages. His gardening activities did suffer some, but not enough to be very noticeable to anyone but him. He just aimed his efforts at plants that required minimum care, spending the rest of the time with Ada.

He had worked a long time as an independent writer, and over the years had worked out a work routine of writing early for five or six hours and then doing something that was a diversion. Many times he would wake up at 04:00, his mind would turn on, and he would get up and start writing, sustained by a cup of coffee and an instant breakfast. Then would come a light lunch, followed by a short nap, and then diversion activity. Before Ada the diversions had been gardening, a self developed exercise and walking program, and reading, with watching videos filling in when he was more tired—it was easy to sleep on a video. Now Ada took up most of his diversionary time, with gardening filling in where time was available. Jake still worked at his exercise program, but not on as routine of a schedule as before Ada. And it was true that much of his diversionary time was spent with Ada sharing the same activities that he had done before—except for the love-making. That was an added attraction.

This clandestine relationship continued in this manner for almost a year.

- - -

Mike left Friday evening to go deer hunting at his lease over near Bracketville. He hadn't been on his stand for an hour Saturday morning when he had already killed his two-buck limit. He field dressed the deer, loaded them into the back of his pick-up, and started home, a day early. He had more than the usual campfire spirit the night before, and had a hell of a headache. He had also had a rough week, and just wanted to get home. He could sleep most of the day Sunday and be back in top form for Monday.

He arrived back in Elmsville early Sunday morning. The processing plant wouldn't be open until about 10:00 when he could drop off the deer. He decided to go home first and get some breakfast and a shower, and then drop off the deer. When he got home, Ada's Camero was in the driveway, but no Ada. Her purse was on the table where she dropped it when she came in, but her keys weren't there. Guess she was out for an early morning walk. He fixed a pot of coffee and some eggs and toast. As he sat in the breakfast area in the kitchen eating, he was looking out over the garden and noted the back gate to the garden was standing open. Mike was just busting with pride over his getting his limit of two deer the first hour of the hunt. He wanted to tell someone about it—to brag a bit—but everyone he knew was out on a hunt themselves ..... except Jake. Jake wasn't much of a hunter himself, but he was worth talking to about the two bucks within an hour. He called Jake, but only got his answering machine. He left a message. He didn't get to talk to anyone, but just talking about the feat to a machine gave him pleasure.

81

Mike went into the bedroom to prepare to take a shower. As he undressed, he noticed that Ada had already made up the bed. He thought, "She must have gotten up early to have already made the bed. She had also cleaned up the kitchen from breakfast—the coffee pot had even been cold, and she always had to have a cup of coffee in the morning to start the day. As he was finishing his shower, he heard the front door slam. "That you, Ada?"

"Yes." She walked into the bedroom area and talked through the open door of the bathroom. "You get anything?

"Yeah, there are two nice bucks in the back of the truck. I'll take them down to the processing plant in a few minutes. I think they open at 10:00. Where have you been?"

"Oh, just out walking. It's such a beautiful morning."

He dressed and was going out through the kitchen. He noted that Ada was dressed in a bright colored shift. "That's a sexy looking outfit to be out walking in so early in the morning."

"It's OK. No one else is out this time on Sunday morning to see me.

Jake was preoccupied thinking about how Ada was dressed, and turned the wrong way when he backed out of the driveway.

"Damn," Mike thought as he realized his mistake and turned into the first side street and came around on the road that ran behind their Garden, between their place and the vacant lots. Mike noticed the back gate to the garden was shut. There was nothing over here on this back street except ..... Jake's place ..... suddenly two plus two added up to four—many small things suddenly fell into place and painted a picture that really infuriated him. "That son-of-a-bitch," Mike thought, "Damn! Damn! Damn!" He acted on impulse and slid his pick-up to a stop in Jake's side driveway. He stormed into Jake's place to confront him.

- - -

All three of them sitting at the table had mentally gone over what had happened among them during the past few months. Mike didn't know when it had started, but reflecting back, he reckoned that it had been going on for some time. Little things began to come back into his conscious memory that he had missed before, all providing bits of supporting evidence that

Ada and Jake had been getting together for some time. He had missed their significance initially. Now they began to pile up.

End Game

Mike was the first to break the silence, "How long has this been going on between you two?"

Jake and Ada looked at each other. It was Jake that spoke, "for a few months now." It was only a partially truthful response. The affair had been going on for a bit more than a year, but Jake didn't see any sense in rubbing Mike's nose in it.

Ada responded, "That's about right." Something they agreed upon without having worked it out in advance.

"And I trusted you!" Mike exclaimed.

Ada responded, "And at one time, I trusted you. Was that violated?"

Mike ignored the question. "Jake, I'm going to get you for this ..... I believe it's called 'alienation of affection'?"

Jake didn't respond. He felt trapped. He knew he was guilty. He still wanted Ada, but the dishonesty of their clandestine relationship made him feel guilty as hell. Jake was basically an honest person, and he had always had trouble defending an action that he knew was wrong.

Ada came to Jake's rescue, "Mike, I'm not sure there was any affection between you and me for Jake to alienate, so don't take it out on him. I was the one that was looking for a little affection."

Mike turned to look at Ada. Fury suddenly exploded across his face. He half rose out of his seat, leaned across the table toward Ada, and at the same time, drew back his right hand as if to start an open-handed slap at Ada's face. "You bitch!"

Mike was greatly surprised at how quick and how strong Jake was. He had reached over and stopped Mike's swing before it had gotten started. Mike just hadn't expected such action from an older man. Jake was still holding Mike's wrist, slightly twisting it counter clockwise toward him. At first Mike didn't quite realize what Jake was doing. He was just shocked that Jake stopped his swing with such seeming ease—actually, Jake had caught the swing just before it started forward, before it had any force. The sudden pain in his elbow pointedly let Mike know that Jake had twisted his arm from the wrist so suddenly that he had gone beyond the point that Mike could use the strength of his arm. Jake moved slightly forward and exerted sudden pressure with the full power of his arm to twist the arm further over. Mike came with the arm as it went, out of his chair and sprawled on the floor. Jake jammed the toes of his right foot into Mike's arm-pit as hard as he could, still holding the extended and twisted arm. Mike screamed in pain. Jake repeated the action. Same results. While still twisting the arm at the wrist, Jake started speaking quietly, "Now let's not get physical. We have a problem here that requires calm deliberation, and passionate physical action will be counter productive. Do you agree to sit quietly and discuss the situation, or do I have to twist some more?"

Mike responded, "OK! OK!"

Jake released his grip, but stood ready to handle any physical challenge that might come from Mike. None came.

Mike picked up his chair with his left hand, holding his right arm close to his side and bent across his stomach, and sat down. He started rubbing his right elbow. He looked at Ada, "I'm sorry Ada. My temper got the best of me. I won't do that again." He looked at Jake, "OK, let's talk, you son-of-a-bitch."

Jake said, "You two are married, and I think you should work out your differences."

Mike exclaimed, "No shit! You really think so? Is that what you were doing—helping us to work out our differences?"

Jake ignored the comment, "I just think you should work out your marriage problems, and everything else will fall into place."

Mike was adamant, "Bullshit! You fuck my wife, and you think we should work out our marriage problem? You're the problem in our marriage!"

Ada got into the shouting match, "No, Mike! Jake wasn't the problem! He was my attempt to find something that you and I had lost! It was my mistake to get him involved!"

The session degenerated into a shouting match—they were all shouting at once, no one listening.

Mike got up from the table, "I'm out of here! This is bullshit! Jake, I'll see you in court! Ada, get your ass home, now!" With that, Mike stormed out the kitchen door, got into his pick-up and threw gravel.

Jake and Ada sat silently for a few moments, just looking at each other.

"Jake, I'm sorry that I got you into this," Ada finally said. "You're right that Mike And I need to get something straightened out in our marriage." She was looking down at the floor now, and continued, "Unfortunately, I chose you as a distraction rather than work on the real problem ....." she looked up at Jake, "..... and I really fell for you. I love you very much, and don't want to see you hurt."

Jake talked softly, "The feeling is mutual ..... I ran into it with my eyes open. I just hope it doesn't splatter on you too badly. I also love you very much."

"Well, I guess it's time for me to go home and face the music," Ada said. With that, she arose, picked up her purse, walked over to Jake and kissed him on the forehead. "Take care, my love."

Jake responded, "Call me. If Mike tries the tough man route again, let me know, quickly."

Jake didn't get up. Ada let herself out and went home.

A little later Jake went over to the counter, picked up the .44, placed it on safety, and stuck it in his belt. He then went back into the utility area, retrieved the pump-gun, and placed it in a closet in the utility area. "I don't think I'll return this to Mike just yet," Jake thought.

- - -

Jake didn't hear from Ada for almost a week. Then it was a telephone call. She said she was doing OK—at least as well as could be expected. She and Mike had some long talks, but as yet nothing was resolved. He hadn't tried physical abuse. They were living in the same house, but were having very little contact. Mike was sleeping in the den. He had contacted a lawyer to pursue the alienation of affection suit. She hoped that Jake was holding up under the pressure. She ended the conversation with, "I love you Jake. Good-bye."

Jake didn't know if that was "good-bye, good-bye" or "good-bye until we talk again." The ambiguity caused him severe emotional anguish.

A New Beginning

Jake decided to leave Elmsville. No matter what happened with the threat by Mike for an alienation of affection lawsuit, he didn't think he could stand to live next door to Ada and not share her life completely. He placed the house in the hands of a real estate agent to sell or lease. The agent was enthusiastic about a sale. She said that the house was in good shape, the market was right, and he had set a fair price. He had arranged to have a moving company come out and pick up the furniture for storage, and they had just completed that job.

Jake had the trailer checked over and serviced by the local RV dealer, and had it in the side driveway loading it in preparation for his next adventure. He actually wasn't feeling too good emotionally. The affair with Ada and its tramatic conclusion had left him emotionally drained. He was somewhat just going through the motions of preparing for an extended trip in the trailer, but he had done it so many times before he wasn't forgetting anything important. Although he was running on empty emotionally, experience, routine, and habit were still working well. He was about ready to pull out, and decided to take one last walk around the inside of the house to reminisce and check for anything he might have forgotten to take care of. He had finished his walk around, locked up the house, and was out on the porch when Ada drove in behind the trailer.

"God, she looks beautiful!" Jake thought. He said, "Hi."

She walked up on the porch. "Hi, Jake. About ready to pull out?"

"Yeah, about ready," Jake lied. He wasn't ready to go at all. He wanted to stay near her, but knew it was impossible.

"Would you like to have a companion on the trip?" she asked. "Before you answer that there are a few things you should know."

Jake was stunned. "What did you say?"

"I asked if you would like to have a companion on your trip. I also said that there are a few things you should know before you answer."

"What?"

"First, don't worry about the lawsuit that Mike threatened. He has changed his mind. He and I are going to get a divorce, uncontested by either of us. I'm free to go with you .....", and she added softly, " ..... and I love you very much."

She was standing a few feet away from Jake. He responded with action rather than words. He leaped toward her, gathered her into his arms and kissed her passionately. She responded in kind. They embraced for some time, just enjoying being held by each other. It was the first time they had touched since that fateful day in the kitchen with Mike.

"When can you be ready to go?" Jake asked her. I was just fixing to pull out."

"I'm ready. My bags are in the back of the Camero. I'll have to drive it back over to Mike's and leave it."

- - -

As Elmsville was receding in the rear view mirror of Jake's truck, Ada was using the middle seat belt, snuggled up beside Jake. Jake put his right arm around her and kissed her on the forehead. "I'm sorry I can't use both hands Ada. Have to drive with one, you know."

93

"By the way Jake, there is one more thing you should have known before you answered so dramatically whether I could go with you .....," she paused, and asked the question, "How do you feel about twelve more years in the PTA?"

"What?"

"I'm pregnant!" After a pause to let that statement sink in and before Jake could recover to respond, she continued, "I'm about two months pregnant. I've known for some time, but couldn't find the right time to tell you. It's your child. Have no fear about that. Mike hasn't touched me for many months. He also doesn't know. I haven't, and won't, tell him until the divorce is final. We have a signed memorandum of understanding, properly witnessed, and signed by us, initialed by both lawyers working the case, and approved by the judge that's involved, but open knowledge of this pregnancy might screw things up. For the time being, it's our secret."

Again, Jake responded by action rather than words. He pulled off on the shoulder of the road, placed the truck in park, and turned to Ada. "For this I'm going to need both hands." He reached over and unbuckled her seat belt, turned her to face him, and kissed her passionately. She kissed back.

It was some time before Jake started driving again, and after a short time he said, there's a state recreation area a few miles east of this next intersection that has a beautiful river front and a trailer park with full utilities. What do you say we park the trailer there for a few days?

She didn't answer in words this time. She just smiled, kissed him and snuggled up.

- - -

During the next few days Ada confided to Jake the events that led up to her being able to leave with him and Mike agreeing not to push the alienation of affection lawsuit. Ada had received a telephone call from an acquaintance that worked with Mike.

"Ada, you may not remember me, Della Burns? I was a couple of years behind you in high school, and I work with Mike.

"Yes, Della. I remember you."

"I understand that you and Mike are having marital problems."

"Yes, we are," Ada admitted. She thought, "The grapevine is already humming!"

"I think we should talk. It will be worth your while. What about lunch at the Inn in about an hour?"

"Fine, I'll be there." Ada was mentally occupied with what to do to straighten out her life, and wondered why she had agreed to do lunch, but she showed up, and on time. It was most fortunate that she did.

- - -

Ada summarized what had happened to make things work out in their favor. She had contacted a private investigator, provided him with some rough, general information—generally what she had received as gossip from Della Burns—about the investigation she proposed, and dropped the requested retainer fee. A week later she had the investigator's report, and documented evidence concerning what she was looking for. She had conferred with her attorney, he agreed with her proposed line of action, and they had arranged a meeting with Mike and his attorney.

At the meeting she informed Mike she was filing suit for divorce on the grounds of long-term adultery, and maintenance support of $2,000 a month. Mike started to laugh off her threat, until she showed him and his attorney a copy of the investigator's report and copies of the supporting documentation, including pictures. After all that had sunk in, she offered an alternative: If Mike would drop the planned alienation suit against Jake, agree to an uncontested divorce, and they split everything right down the middle, she would drop the adultery suit. Mike and his lawyer walked outside and conferred a few minutes. When they came back in, Mike said it was a deal. Her lawyer handed Mike's lawyer a drafted memorandum of understanding containing the elements of Ada's proposal, and they went to see the judge. It all worked out. No one except the two lawyers and Ada and Mike saw the investigator's report or the supporting documents. The supporting documents were sworn statements by a widow that was one of Mike's customers and a waitress over in Hopdale indicating Mike had been having sexual relations with them on a rather routine basis for three and over four years respectfully—and there were pictures of Mike meeting the two ladies at places he was not supposed to have been. The agreement with these women was that there would be no messy alienation of affection law-suits brought against them by Ada, with the accompanying bad publicity, and Ada would only use the documents if absolutely necessary in a divorce case against Mike. Needless to say, Mike was caught with his pants down, literally. Ada's threat balanced Mike's threat—on advice of counsel they called it a draw, and agreed to split the blanket and go their separate ways. Ada had chosen to go with Jake. It proved to be a good choice.

Ada confided in Jake that she had decided to have the baby and raise her or him even before she had told Jake she was pregnant. She was ready to raise the baby herself as a single parent if Jake wasn't interested in playing the fatherhood bit again. "If He is going to give me a second chance at motherhood, I sure as hell am going to take full advantage of the opportunity, and do everything in my power to do it right," is the way she put it. "I was going to go with you to love you as long as I could, and if you didn't want to be a father, I was going to split, and have a go at it on my own."

Jake put his arms around Ada, and said, "I always wanted another crack at those teachers who didn't think my child was near perfect, and with you there beside me, we should have a blast!"

- - -

Seven months and three days after Ada left Elmsville and after Ada and Mike's divorce was final, Mike received an announcement:

> Name: Janice Megen Mechem
> Date of Birth: August 4, 1995
> Weight and Height: 8 pounds, 6 ounces. 19.2 inches.
> By: Jake
> Out of: Ada
> A fine filly!

Mike exclaimed, "Well I'll be damned!" when he read it. He did a quick bit of mental mathematical calculation, and again exclaimed, "Well I'll be damned!"

- - -

Informational articles available to those who accessed the local high school computer net, "What's Happening Here at Newtonville Hi," for the school year 2014-2015 proclaimed that Janice Mechem, an honor student, was elected to be the new member of the Varsity Cheerleader Squad; that Jake Mechem, president of the PTA, had received critical acclaim for his semi-autobiographical novel *One More Time*; and that Mrs. Ada Mechem was one of two parent sponsors of the Varsity Cheerleader Squad.

About the Author

T. F. "Jack" Jackson, Jr. grew up first on a Northwest Arkansas cotton plantation at Number 9 and later in Morehouse, a small Southeast Missouri town. He enlisted in the Air Force as a private during the Korean Police Action and stayed on for thirty-three and one-half years, retiring as a Colonel in 1984. While in the Air Force he completed his BS and MBA degrees. After a follow-on stint as a civilian hospital administrator, he decided to continue his education and enrolled in a doctoral program at Texas A&M University, graduating in 1993 earning an Ed D in education with a major in human resources development and minors in management and educational computer technology. It was during the preparation of his dissertation that he decided he might be able to write, a long time secret ambition. Several manuscripts later he is still at it. Now in "retired status" he spends his time reading, writing, gardening, and volunteering for the Bexar County Master Gardeners and the Master Naturalists. He resides in the San Antonio, TX, area and has been married to his childhood sweetheart for almost forty-nine years. They have four sons.

www.ingramcontent.com/pod-product-compliance
Lightning Source LLC
Chambersburg PA
CBHW030354290526
45785CB00004B/1743